Cambridge **Discovery Education**™

► **INTERACTIVE READERS**

Series editor: Bob Hastings

GET SMART
OUR AMAZING BRAIN

GW00759891

B1

Caroline Shackleton and Nathan Paul Turner

CAMBRIDGE
UNIVERSITY PRESS

DISCOVERY
EDUCATION™

CAMBRIDGE
UNIVERSITY PRESS

University Printing House, Cambridge CB2 8BS, United Kingdom

One Liberty Plaza, 20th Floor, New York, NY 10006, USA

477 Williamstown Road, Port Melbourne, VIC 3207, Australia

4843/24, 2nd Floor, Ansari Road, Daryaganj, Delhi – 110002, India

79 Anson Road, #06–04/06, Singapore 079906

Cambridge University Press is part of the University of Cambridge.

It furthers the University's mission by disseminating knowledge in the pursuit of education, learning and research at the highest international levels of excellence.

www.cambridge.org
Information on this title: www.cambridge.org/9781107650633

First published 2014
20 19 18 17 16 15 14 13 12 11 10 9

Printed in Dubai by Oriental Press

A catalogue record for this publication is available from the British Library

Library of Congress Cataloging-in-Publication Data

Shackleton, Caroline.
    Get smart: our amazing brain / Caroline Shackleton and Nathan Paul Turner.
        pages cm. — (Cambridge discovery interactive readers)
    ISBN 978-1-107-65063-3 (pbk. : alk. paper)
1. Brain—Juvenile literature. 2. English language—Textbooks for foreign speakers.
3. Readers (Elementary) I. Title.

QP376.S4372 2013
612.8'2—dc23

                            2013025121

ISBN 978-1-107-65063-3

Additional resources for this publication at www.cambridge.org

Layout services, art direction, book design, and photo research: Q2ABillSMITH GROUP
Editorial services: Hyphen S.A.
Audio production: CityVox, New York
Video production: Q2ABillSMITH GROUP

Contents

Before You Read: Get Ready!

Words to Know

Read the article. Then complete the definitions with the correct highlighted words.

The human brain is more powerful than the fastest supercomputer. It controls all your body's processes, from your heartbeat to your sense of balance. It is also where your feelings and emotions and your conscious thoughts and decisions take place.

Our brain has about 100 billion electrical connections, called neurons, or brain cells, which send and receive information from the body and help us understand our world. If the brain is hurt, our movement, senses, and even our personality can suffer. But the brain is very flexible. It is constantly changing and growing and can often redirect neural connections when damaged. By studying the problems of people with brain damage, scientists have learned a lot about the brain's functions.

1. _____: the smallest parts of the brain, which send messages to other parts of the body
2. _____: the jobs that things do
3. _____: actions or changes that happen naturally
4. _____: awake and able to think
5. _____: the ability to stop yourself from falling over
6. _____: hurt or injured
7. _____: what makes each of us different
8. _____: feelings such as love or anger
9. _____: able to change or be changed easily

Look at the drawing of the brain and the definitions. As you read about different parts of the brain, use this information to help you understand where they are located and what they do.

amygdala: a small part of the brain deep inside the temporal lobe that helps produce emotions and memories

brain stem: connects the brain to the rest of the body and controls things people do without thinking, such as breathing

cerebellum: the oldest part of the brain that controls basic movement, and feelings such as fear

cerebrum: the largest part of the brain that controls thinking and movement

cortex: the outer part of the cerebrum and cerebellum made up of gray matter

gray and white matter: two types of matter that make up the cerebrum. The white matter is made up of special cells that carry messages between the cells in the gray matter.

hemispheres: the right and left parts of the cerebrum that often work together to do things such as processing language

lobes: the four main areas of the brain

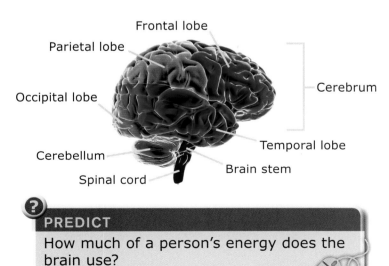

PREDICT

How much of a person's energy does the brain use?

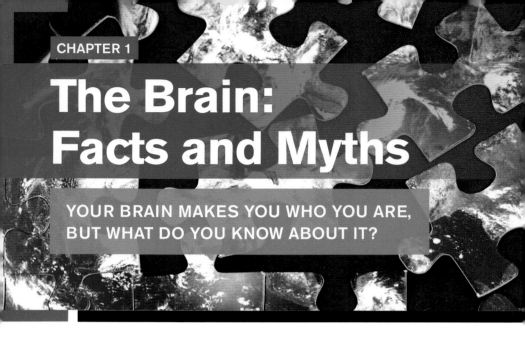

CHAPTER 1

The Brain: Facts and Myths

YOUR BRAIN MAKES YOU WHO YOU ARE,
BUT WHAT DO YOU KNOW ABOUT IT?

In the past, people knew little about the human brain. The Greek philosopher Aristotle believed we thought with our hearts! Now, thanks to science, we know more. But what do *you* know about your brain?

Read the sentences. Decide whether each one is a fact (true) or **myth** (not true).

1. People only use about 10 percent of the brain.
   Fact / Myth

2. People use one hemisphere of the brain more than the other.
   Fact / Myth

3. Once **brain cells** die, new ones cannot grow in their place.
   Fact / Myth

4. The brain, like a computer, has a fixed and limited[1] memory.
   Fact / Myth

....

[1] **limited:** has an amount that can't be changed

5. The white matter in the brain doesn't do anything important.
Fact / Myth

6. The brain uses almost a quarter of all a person's energy.
Fact / Myth

7. Teenage brains aren't totally finished **developing**.
Fact / Myth

8. Men and women think differently.
Fact / Myth

9. The brain can repair itself after an accident.
Fact / Myth

10. The different lobes in the brain do different jobs.
Fact / Myth

The Answers

1. Myth. We use different parts of the brain at different times and for different functions, so we really use a large amount of our brain. In fact, if neurons aren't used, they die.

2. Myth. Until recently, many scientists believed that people used one half of the brain more than the other. Now we know the brain uses both sides together. For example, while the left side processes language, the right side controls the way we speak.

3. Myth. Many people think that as we get older, our brain cells die away, making us less intelligent. Fortunately, adults can grow new neurons by learning new things, doing exercise, and remembering things.

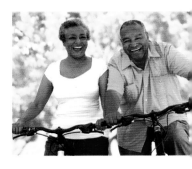

4. Myth. When we remember something, our brain is actually making new memory connections for the first time!

5. Myth. In the past, scientists thought that white matter didn't do anything important. Now they know that it is full of special cells, called glia, which help control the neural signals and also clean and repair neuron cells.

6. Fact. Our brain uses about 20 percent of all our energy and 25 percent of all the oxygen we breathe.

7. Fact. Studies show that teenagers don't use as much of the brain as adults. In particular, the frontal lobe, which controls social feelings and guilt, is less active. In other words, teenagers really are more selfish than adults! However, the brain becomes fully adult by about age 17.

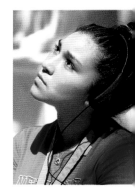

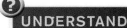

UNDERSTAND
How has our understanding about how the brain works changed?

8. Myth. Although it is true that men's and women's brains have different amounts of white and gray matter, new studies show that there seems to be no difference between how well men and women think and solve problems.

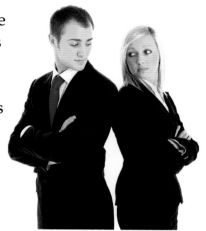

9. Fact. The brain is actually very flexible. When a part of the brain is damaged, other parts of the brain often **create** new connections to do the job of the missing part.

10. Fact. With the frontal lobe we think, plan, and feel emotion. With the parietal lobe we taste things and feel touch, pressure,[2] pain, or temperature. The occipital lobe lets us see the world. The temporal lobe lets us hear things, and it is also important for emotion and memory.

[2]**pressure:** the feeling when you push something

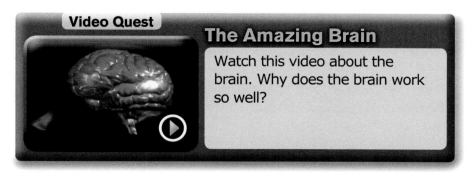

Video Quest

The Amazing Brain

Watch this video about the brain. Why does the brain work so well?

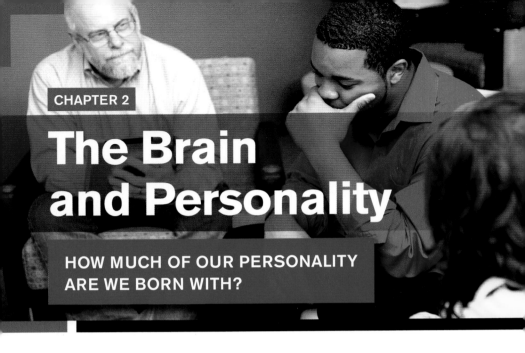

CHAPTER 2

The Brain and Personality

HOW MUCH OF OUR PERSONALITY ARE WE BORN WITH?

What type of personality do you have? Are you shy or outgoing, cheerful or sad? Many psychologists[3] **divide** human personality into these five general personality types:

- Extrovert – how outgoing and social we are

- Neurotic – how angry, guilty, or worried we are

- Agreeable – how kind, friendly, and trusting[4] we are

- Conscientious – how self-controlled, responsible, and organized we are

- Open – how interested in new things we are

Psychologists see our personalities as a mix of different amounts of each type. They use personality tests – special lists of questions – to decide how much of each type a person has.

[3]**psychologist:** a person who studies the human mind and feelings
[4]**trusting:** believing people are good and honest

But how much of a person's personality is learned from other people, and how much are people born with? And are the five types connected to different parts of the brain?

In the 1980s, studies were carried out on identical twins (born from the same egg) who had grown up with different families. Although the children often grew up in very different places with different people, scientists found that they usually had extremely similar personalities. These studies led the scientists to realize that our brain controls our behavior and personality much more than they had previously thought.

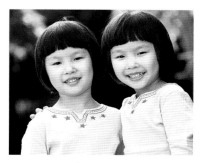

Scientists study identical twins to learn about personality.

Today, scientists have the technology to take a computer picture, or scan, that shows which areas of the brain are being used when

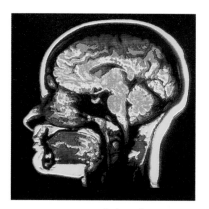

A brain scan

people think, speak, and act. This means they can look for connections between the scans and the results of traditional personality tests. The results are both interesting and **complicated**.

So what is the exact relationship between personality and the areas of the brain?

Certain areas of the brain seem to be stronger in different people, depending on their personality. Brain scans of strongly extroverted people show them to have a larger frontal lobe than shy people. The frontal lobe controls social functions in humans and also helps give feelings of pleasure. So, outgoing people enjoy group situations like parties, and they like being given compliments[5] and getting prizes.

In fact, a new study found that four of the five main personality types have a direct relationship to the size of different areas in the brain. People who are more responsible, who worry more, and those who are friendlier all have more neuron connections in specific areas!

[5]**compliment:** something nice that is said or written about somebody

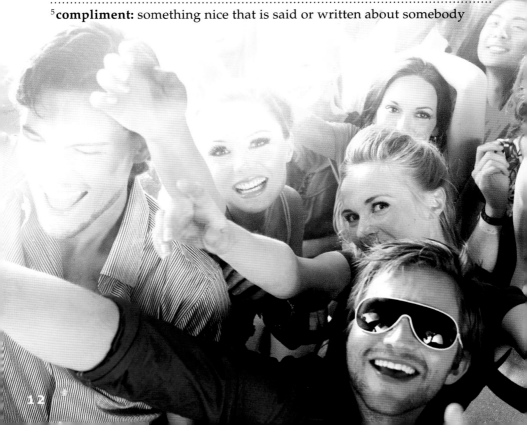

The only personality type that seems to have no clear connection to a physical part of the brain is how open we are to new experiences and information.

Does this mean that a personality can't be changed? Not at all! In fact, scientists now know the brain is very flexible. Often, functions are shared by different parts of the brain.

What's more, doing something like playing a musical instrument will make the brain grow more neurons in the area being used. This means that when one type of behavior is repeated, like being sociable, that tells the brain to **produce** more neurons, helping someone do that behavior better.

So, if you want to be more organized, try making small changes, like always putting your keys in the same place, or studying at the same time every day. If you want to be more outgoing, try taking part in social activities. The more you talk to people, the more this part of your brain will respond!

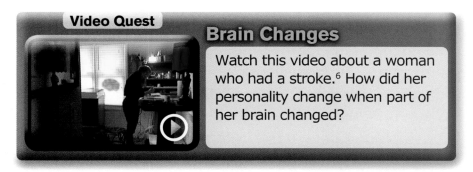

Video Quest

Brain Changes

Watch this video about a woman who had a stroke.[6] How did her personality change when part of her brain changed?

[6]**stroke:** an illness caused by a change in the amount of blood reaching the brain

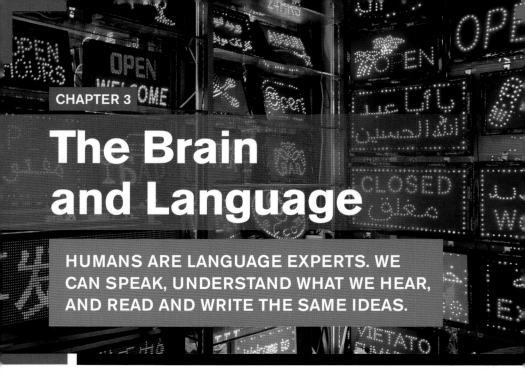

CHAPTER 3

The Brain and Language

HUMANS ARE LANGUAGE EXPERTS. WE CAN SPEAK, UNDERSTAND WHAT WE HEAR, AND READ AND WRITE THE SAME IDEAS.

Many scientists believe that language is the one ability that really separates humans from other animals. While many other animals, such as chimpanzees and dolphins, live in groups and communicate, scientists don't know for certain whether they can talk and share complicated ideas.

How does the brain **deal with** language? For most people, the main language center is in the left hemisphere. However, for about 19 percent of people who are left-handed, the main language center is in the right hemisphere, and as many as 68 percent of left-handed people use both parts equally. In fact, everybody uses a little of both hemispheres for language. If the stronger hemisphere is damaged, language ability can develop in the other.

In the 19th century, scientists began to study patients with *aphasia*. Aphasia is an inability to speak or understand language that results from brain damage, usually because of an accident. Although scientists at that time didn't have brain scans to show them which areas of the brain were damaged, this information was usually clear from the patient's accident.

Scientists discovered two important language areas in the brain. The first, Broca's area, toward the front of the brain, was thought to produce speech. People with a damaged Broca's area could understand language but couldn't speak.

The second, Wernicke's area, toward the back of the brain, seemed to do the opposite. People with Wernicke's aphasia cannot understand others. They can speak, but it is a mix of words without meaning.

Scientists learned that the first area was important for producing language and the second for understanding it.

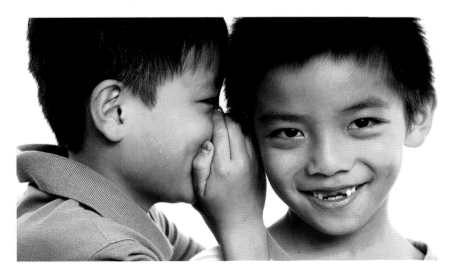

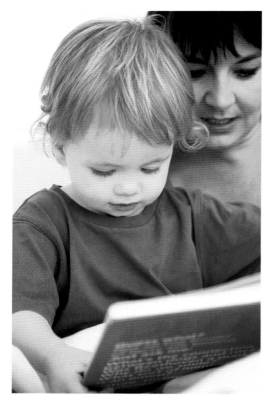

Much more recently, in 2005, new brain scan technology let scientists see the nerve connections between the two areas in much more detail. This led them to the discovery of a third area, known as Geschwind's area. It connects Broca's and Wernicke's areas. It seems to be the last area to develop in the brain and may develop in children as they learn language.

How does the brain learn language? Everyone knows children are the best language learners. In fact, babies have twice as many neurons as adults. But, although at first babies have the ability to hear and learn all human sounds, they soon start to choose only the ones that they hear being spoken around them.

Their ability to learn language easily seems to disappear around the age of twelve. After this age, learning to speak for the first time becomes almost impossible, and even learning a second language becomes more difficult.

People who speak two languages very well are called bilingual. Today, it is thought that more than half the people living in the world are bilingual. In many countries the large number of different societies and nationalities means that people *must* speak at least two languages.

Where do bilingual brains store[7] languages? Some scientists think that bilingual people store different languages in different parts of the brain. Bilingual people with brain damage to one part of the brain often lose the ability to speak one language but not the other.

Recently, scientists have learned that bilingual people develop more gray matter than people who only speak one language, which may make their brains stronger in the case of an accident or a health problem. So, speaking a second language is not only useful, it may also be healthy!

[7]**store:** keep something somewhere until it is needed

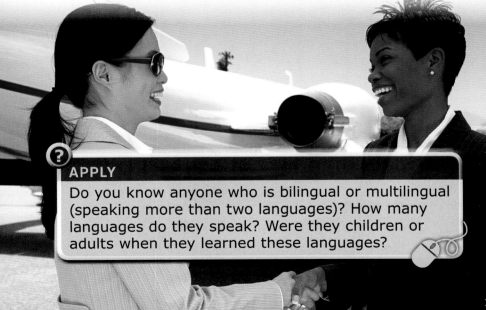

APPLY

Do you know anyone who is bilingual or multilingual (speaking more than two languages)? How many languages do they speak? Were they children or adults when they learned these languages?

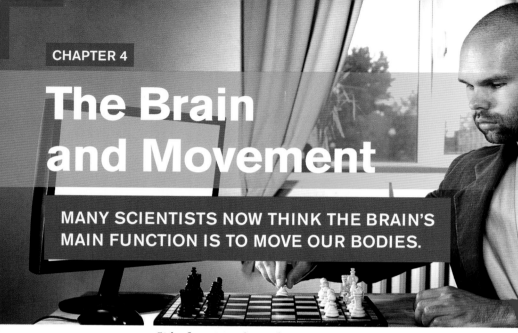

CHAPTER 4

The Brain and Movement

MANY SCIENTISTS NOW THINK THE BRAIN'S MAIN FUNCTION IS TO MOVE OUR BODIES.

It's fun to play chess against a computer.

Movement may seem like a simple thing, but it's actually more complicated than the "higher skills" of language and thought. One brain scientist said that, although we can make a computer that can beat world champions at chess, we still can't make a robot that can move nearly as well as us.

Have you ever tried to tickle yourself? It's almost impossible. Because the brain knows what is going to happen, you don't feel it in the same way. Our own touch doesn't make us laugh or move away from the tickling fingers.

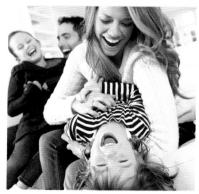

We can't tickle ourselves.

Movement uses many areas of the brain. It is a complicated process of balance, muscle control, and prediction. The brain makes it look easy, but there's still a lot we don't know about it.

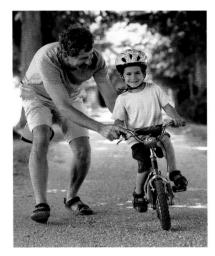

By the 1960s, brain scientists had found that they could make **muscles** move by sending electrical signals to the motor cortex, the part of the cortex that deals with movement. In their experiments, scientists found that the motor cortex has areas of gray matter for each of the body's 650 different muscles.

The largest part of the motor cortex is used to control the hands. Although your hands are not the biggest part of your body, they need much more brain power because they make very complicated movements!

The motor cortex controls conscious movements, but there are many other movements that people do unconsciously. Balance, for example, is controlled by the cerebellum. And the brain stem controls things people do without even thinking, like breathing.

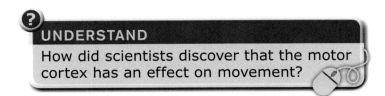

?
UNDERSTAND
How did scientists discover that the motor cortex has an effect on movement?

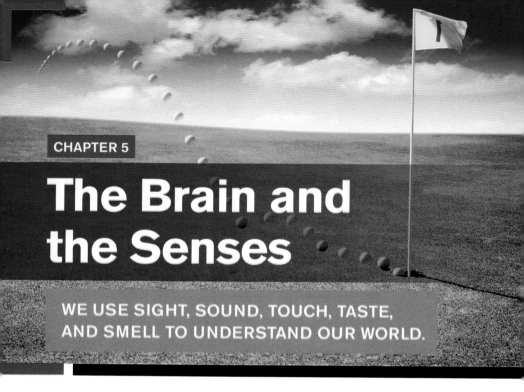

CHAPTER 5

The Brain and the Senses

WE USE SIGHT, SOUND, TOUCH, TASTE, AND SMELL TO UNDERSTAND OUR WORLD.

Of course there is no point in being able to move if you don't know where you are going or what you're doing! To understand the information our senses give us, we use our brains. Let's look at how our brains control the senses.

Sight

Sight is actually a set of very complicated systems. When you watch a ball flying through the air, the color information and the movement information sent from the eyes are being read by different parts of the brain at the same time. Although most of the information goes to the visual cortex, which processes sight information, some of the eye's nerves send information to the cerebellum, too, which helps control balance and movement. This means you can catch the ball, too!

Because different parts of the brain read different information about what we see, damage to the brain can change what and how we see. *Akinetopsia*, for example, is an illness where a person cannot see movement. For these people, life is like looking at the world in photos! A person with akinetopsia can't see the movement of water, for example. So, he might use hearing to help fill a glass.

Smell

The main olfactory nerve, which sends smell information, is the fastest in the brain. The speed of smell is faster than the speed of light or sound! Our sense of smell is very powerful – it can even make us feel sick!

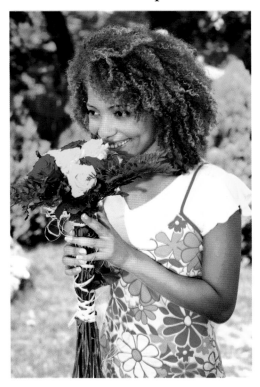

Because smell is connected to the temporal lobe, which helps us store memories, particular smells can also bring up very particular memories. In fact, people can easily remember as many as 10,400 smells!

Sound

The sound of a knife on a plate or fingernails on a chalkboard can be really annoying. But why is that? It's because high sounds like those go to the part of the brain called the amygdala, which creates emotions. Other sounds, like music, are processed in the reward center of the brain and give us pleasure.

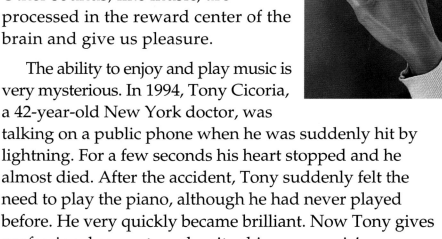

The ability to enjoy and play music is very mysterious. In 1994, Tony Cicoria, a 42-year-old New York doctor, was talking on a public phone when he was suddenly hit by lightning. For a few seconds his heart stopped and he almost died. After the accident, Tony suddenly felt the need to play the piano, although he had never played before. He very quickly became brilliant. Now Tony gives professional concerts and writes his own music!

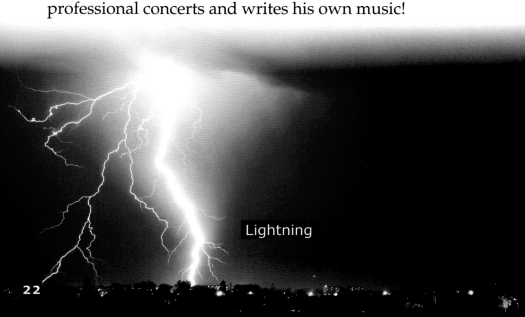

Lightning

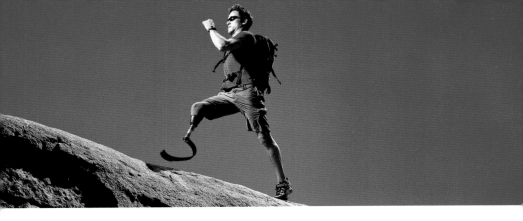

Feeling

When you hit your toe, it feels like the pain is in your toe. In fact, it isn't. The pain is a message from your brain. This is why many people who have lost an arm or leg in an accident can still feel the limb.[8] They even report that they can still feel pain in the lost limb!

A few people have a different and extremely rare problem: they feel no pain. This may sound great, but it can be very dangerous, especially in children. Feeling no pain also means they don't know when they are hurting themselves. One girl bit off her own tongue while eating and regularly burned herself because she couldn't feel heat or even electric shocks.

[8]**limb:** an arm or a leg
[9]**epileptic seizure:** an electrical problem in the brain

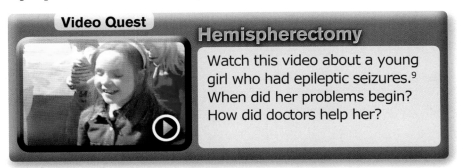

Video Quest

Hemispherectomy

Watch this video about a young girl who had epileptic seizures.[9] When did her problems begin? How did doctors help her?

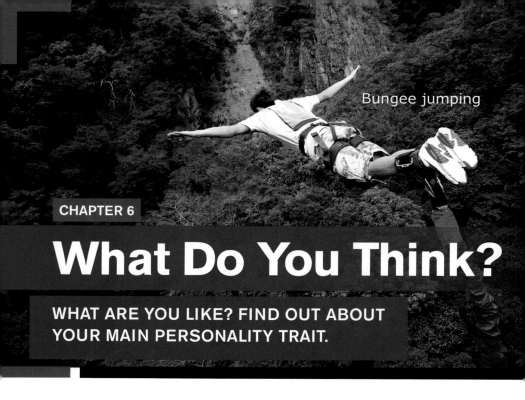

Bungee jumping

CHAPTER 6

What Do You Think?

WHAT ARE YOU LIKE? FIND OUT ABOUT YOUR MAIN PERSONALITY TRAIT.

Take the quiz and choose the best answer for you.

1 When I go to a party, _____ .
- (A) I love talking to new people
- (B) I help clean up afterwards
- (C) I help organize the food and drinks
- (D) I organize party games

2 In my free time I prefer to _____ .
- (A) go out with friends
- (B) help my friends and family
- (C) study
- (D) go to a museum or art gallery

3 My favorite sport or exercise is _____ .
- (A) a team sport with my friends, like soccer
- (B) whatever everyone else wants to do
- (C) going to the gym on my own
- (D) something new or adventurous, like bungee jumping

4 I organize my time _____.

   (A) to be with other people

   (B) depending on what other people want to do

   (C) very well (everything is planned)

   (D) to do many different things

5 My room is _____.

   (A) always full of people

   (B) never locked

   (C) always clean and tidy

   (D) original and designed by me

6 My friends describe me most often as _____.

   (A) outgoing

   (B) a good friend

   (C) organized

   (D) **creative**

7 When I receive an unexpected but interesting invitation, I _____.

   (A) ask how many people will be there

   (B) cancel or change my plans and accept

   (C) check my calendar before accepting

   (D) accept it immediately

8 My plans for the future are _____.

   (A) to travel around the world and meet lots of people

   (B) to help others as much as possible

   (C) to study a lot and get a good job

   (D) to do lots of different things

....

Mostly A's: You have an extroverted personality.

Mostly B's: You have an agreeable personality.

Mostly C's: You have a conscientious personality.

Mostly D's: You have an open personality.

After You Read

Read the questions and choose Ⓐ, Ⓑ, Ⓒ, or Ⓓ.

1 How have scientists used computer scans?
- Ⓐ To study personality traits
- Ⓑ To discover if people are twins
- Ⓒ To change people's personalities
- Ⓓ To see how intelligent people are

2 Which part of the brain is associated with sociable people?
- Ⓐ neurons
- Ⓑ frontal lobe
- Ⓒ right hemisphere
- Ⓓ left hemisphere

3 Which two things does Geschwind's area connect?
- Ⓐ white matter and gray matter
- Ⓑ Broca's area and Wernicke's area
- Ⓒ the visual cortex and the cerebellum
- Ⓓ the amygdala and the reward center

4 According to many scientists, what is the brain's main function?
- Ⓐ To smell the world around us
- Ⓑ To create interesting thoughts
- Ⓒ To control our movements
- Ⓓ To show others our intelligence

5 Which part of the brain allows us to move without falling over?
- Ⓐ the brain stem
- Ⓑ the motor cortex
- Ⓒ the cerebrum
- Ⓓ the cerebellum

6 Which sense helps most with memories?

- (A) sight
- (B) smell
- (C) sound
- (D) touch

7 Why do people dislike some noises?

- (A) Because they make feelings happen in the brain
- (B) Because they kill some brain cells
- (C) Because they are processed in the reward center
- (D) Because the imagination reacts badly

True or False?

Read the sentences and choose T (true) or F (false).

1 We don't use some of the neurons in our brain.   T/F

2 New brain cells grow because of activity.   T/F

3 Extroverted people like rewards.   T/F

4 It is thought that an open personality is not shown by the brain.   T/F

5 It is impossible to change your personality.   T/F

6 In the 19th century scientists discovered which parts of
the brain relate to language.   T/F

7 People who speak two languages have more white matter in
their brains.   T/F

8 All the nerves from your eyes go to the visual cortex.   T/F

9 Scientists understand how music is processed in the brain.   T/F

Think About It

Imagine that you were in an accident and hurt your head. You're fine now, but you can no longer feel pain. How would this affect your life? Think of three things that would be easier or better, and three things that would be harder or more dangerous.

Answer Key

Words to Know, page 4
1 neurons **2** functions **3** processes **4** conscious
5 balance **6** damaged **7** personality **8** emotions
9 flexible

Predict, page 5
Answers will vary.

Understand, page 8
We know that one side of the brain is not dominant. Both sides are used together.

Video Quest, page 9
Because neurons communicate with each other.

Video Quest, page 13
She became more visual, imaginative, and emotional. She was more artistic.

Apply, page 17
Answers will vary.

Understand, page 19
By sending electrical signals to different areas of the brain.

Video Quest, page 23
Six weeks after her third birthday. They removed her right hemisphere.

Choose the Correct Answers, page 26
1 A **2** B **3** B **4** C **5** D **6** B **7** A

True or False, page 27
1 F **2** T **3** T **4** T **5** F **6** T **7** F **8** F **9** F

Think about it, page 27
Answers will vary.